Legal & Disclaimer

The information contained in this book is not designed to replace or take the place of any form of medication or professional medical advice. The information in this book has been provided for educational and entertainment purposes only.

The information contained in this book has been compiled from sources deemed reliable, and it is accurate to the best of the Author's knowledge. However, the Author cannot guarantee its accuracy and validity so cannot be held liable for any errors or omissions. Changes are periodically made to this book. You must consult your doctor or get professional medical advice before using any of the suggested remedies, techniques, or information in this book.

Upon using the information contained in this book, you agree to hold harmless the Author from and against any damages, costs and expenses, including any legal fees, potentially resulting from the application of any of the information provided by this guide. This disclaimer applies to any damages or injury caused by the use and application, whether directly or indirectly, of any advice or information presented, whether for breach of contract, tort, negligence, personal injury, criminal intent, or under any other cause of action.

You agree to accept all the risks of using the information presented inside this book. You need to consult a professional medical practitioner in order to ensure you are both able & healthy enough to participate in this program.

Contents

Chapter 1: The Triad of Health 3

    Nutrition 4

    Exercise 4

    Mental Conditioning 5

Chapter 2: Mindfulness Exercise 7

Chapter 3: Eat Less, Eat Frequently, Eat Regularly 9

Chapter 4: Check the Label 11

Chapter 5: Goodbye Gadgets... 13

Chapter 6: Emptying the Stash 15

Chapter 7: Don't Give in to Stress 17

Chapter 8: Hit the Kitchen 19

Chapter 9: Walk, Walk, Walk... 21

Conclusion 22

Check Out Other Books 23

Chapter 1: The Triad of Health

It's 6 AM, and you're late for work. You rush to the bathroom and soak in that warm and gentle rain. Your gaze turns towards the big bump in your middle, and you wish you could see your feet. Drying yourself, you look in the mirror, and you notice botches of stretch marks appearing where they shouldn't be. You wear your formal suit, and you realize they're two sizes shorter despite getting them at last month's sale. You struggle to get those pants up and putting those clasps together feels like a corset choking you. You rush to the streets, joining the milieu of people trudging towards morning traffic. After precious minutes of waiting in line, you try walking to a different stop, but you keep taking breaks so you could catch your breath. After hailing a cab, you try to compose yourself for today's meeting, at times opening a button or two to ease up the belly. You arrive at the office, and the elevator is full. The only way you can attend the morning's important meeting in time is to walk the stairs to the third floor. By the time you get to the second, you're whizzing and panting, your whole body disheveled beyond recognition. You go through your day, sometimes feeling a bit dizzy or light-headed, and you realize it's because of that darn button keeping your stomach and dignity confined. Oxygen levels are low, and stress levels are high. It's a good thing there's dinner, and you can reward yourself with extra cups of rice, and juicy portions of roasted pig. You feel a little guilty, so you swig it down with yogurt or order some vegetable side dishes. You end the day in bed, and you promise yourself that tomorrow, tomorrow will be the day you will start your diet. And this is what you tell yourself every night.

Familiar? Losing weight seems to be an emerging problem for everyone, whether you're in the workforce, or you're staying at home, whether you're male or female, young or old. Weight affects all facets of our self-concept, from our perception of our beauty or health. We regularly compare ourselves with others; thinking how everybody else in the social media looks good. Advertisements have made sure you're hooked into the comparison game. You feel that you are not achieving your potential and you wish you could walk faster, move quicker or party harder. Losing weight is at the back of everyone's minds.

There are a lot of health programs out there which are nothing but marketing strategies aimed at weight reduction instantly while robbing you big time. Some work, some don't, and it's an ongoing battle of science and advertising. These programs fall into three particular categories: nutrition, exercise, and mental conditioning. I will illustrate the value of these three programs; why they are popular and time deficient.

Nutrition

A lot of programs emphasize diet. Fats are the consequence of eating more, and these programs go to the core of the matter by monitoring the food intake. Many of these programs have a complicated set of instructions for understanding how nutrition works. But in a nutshell, we say that food and its intake is very important for any program if you want to lose weight. Food supplies the body with the required nutrients to perform its function. Our body is composed of four building blocks: lipids, carbohydrates, nucleic acids, and proteins. The variety of food supplies these basic building blocks, replenishing depleted sources to sustain our activities such as breathing, talking, sleeping to more complicated functions like thinking, planning, organizing. Rice and bread, for example, supply our main carbohydrate source, as well as all the sweets we take in. We need some form of lipids found in oil or animal fat to keep our skin supple and the cell membranes intact. Meat and seafood provide us with nucleic acids and proteins needed for regenerating dead cells and building muscles for movement.

Any program that advocates weight loss will have to consider nutrition. If you think you can just lose weight by thinking about losing weight without proper diet, then you are fooling yourself. You need to observe the changes in your body. You cannot just go to the gym and exercise all you want, hoping to lose weight without acknowledging the need for the proper diet. You can pump all you want, but if at the end of each gym session, you still gobble down two cups of rice, washed down with soda, and then your exercise becomes useless.

But if we only consider diet without the other components, we can still achieve some results, but it will not be optimal. For example, if your nutritionist tells you to eat vegetables or to cut down on carbs, you can effortlessly do this in a week. But your mind can play tricks on you, and you may lose the determination to diet if you solely focus on the food. Or you may think that you can lose weight by just dieting and neglect exercising, and then you could get frustrated with the results. Yes, you will lose some weight but only gradually, and won't become shaped or toned as you want. So the diet is necessary for the better framework of health.

Exercise

Exercise is very significant for any weight loss program. By exercising, you are converting the food into energy. Your fat is burned by exercising, and the activity has a lot of health benefits from blood circulation to better respiration. Exercise tells you that your body is alive and functioning.

However, the truth of our busy lives is that there is no time to hit the gym regularly. There will be periods of motivation; to workout on the machines or enroll in a yoga program. But as the work piles up, we tend to move exercise to a lower priority on the list. This is understandable, and we don't need to punish ourselves for it. But should not give up the fight too. Also, some of these programs cost a lot. A gym membership can extort a scandalous amount from you that is wasted because of your schedule. You may not lose weight, but you are definitely losing money.

The point of all this is that you should move. Sitting all day at the desk while eating the proper kind of food will not be enough to make you lose weight. You have to move, so your blood can circulate and deliver all the nutrients that rest of the body needs. Moving takes away the toxins from your bodies that accumulate and distress you or become a source of diseases. We should always be conscious of moving our body because the principle of atrophy is that whatever we don't use loses function. This is especially true for old people who do not try to walk and are dependent on wheelchairs when they still can walk. If they do not use their feet, they lose the ability to walk. This is the same with normal and healthy individuals in the prime of their lives. If we don't move, we lose functionality.

Mental Conditioning

But can diet and exercise alone reduce weight? Yes, they can. For a few days, or even weeks. If we see weight loss as a condition of the body, then the physical response is appropriate and needed. But can these two alone sustain the weight loss? No, they can't. The problem with dieting and exercising lies in sustaining them. You can eat healthily and jog every day for the next two weeks. But something always comes up to distract you from carrying out your fitness program. Imagine having to eat sweet potato as an alternative to rice or potato chips for the next two days. Sure, it can be healthy. But you will get tired of it, your body will repulse its flavor, or you're going to throw up the next time when you think about eating sweet potatoes.

We need mental conditioning to integrate and sustain any diet or exercise fitness program. This emphasizes the role of the mind in keeping our body healthy. This framework regards health and weight loss not as a physical reality; to be dealt with simple physical solutions. Rather, it recognizes health as a state of mind, as a function of our cognition. Only in this way, our efforts to become fit can be sustainable. The mind is a plastic organ, malleable and trainable. It governs every function in the body and tells us when to take in less or more of our food. Hence, we have to emphasize the role of the mind.

Integrating these three components, I will give you some mini-habits that you can follow to help you reduce weight without the expense and the hassle. I call them 'mini-habits' because they require a small form of change in your life. Many times we feel the drag of making drastic changes in our lifestyle so much that we become disheartened to sustain initial bursts of inspiration. So we will advocate small changes that you can easily do. These are also habits because they should be done on a regular basis. The problem with most fitness or health programs is that they are engaging initially; with people excited to try a new food supplement or a new exercise program. But after a few intakes or a few sessions, they get bored, or other priorities just arise. Sooner or later, they slump back to their old ways. These set of mini-acts are meant to be do-able so you can perform them on a daily basis. After a while, they become automatic, and you become programmed to be healthy. Before engaging in the actual habits, it is good that we understand ourselves and our health goals first. Here is an exercise to guide us through this.

Chapter 2: Mindfulness Exercise

Before starting this exercise, we should be clear about some things first. This is a fitness program for everybody; may or may not have different backgrounds. We have to level the field and assess your readiness for the program. Otherwise, it will be very ineffective, and you will simply achieve sub-optimal results. It is possible to go through the program while bypassing this important step. But you are going to miss a lot of things, and you may find yourself unable to get into some of the exercises as a result.

This exercise will require some time. So find a place now that is quiet enough and that you feel rested. Make sure you don't have any distractions around you. Turn off your cellphones, close your laptops, remove anything that will remind you of your stresses in life. Sit in a comfortable position, but not too relaxing that will make you sleep.

And breathe. Breathe in and out, breathe in and out. Just focus on the air going in your nose, and then out. Breathe in and breath out. Breathe in and breathe out. Imagine all the positive energy going in you, and all the negative energies going out. Breathe in, breath out. Do this for ten minutes.

Slowly, focus your attention on the following questions. Don't rush; just let your stream of consciousness flow without impeding them. If you find yourself distracted, just breathe in and breathe out and then refocus yourself. It is important you feel as relaxed as possible. Slowly, ask yourself:

Do you have things that are holding you back?

Are there things in your life that worry you now? These may be work or family related problems. This may be the bosses you have trouble dealing with, deadlines that are piling up, and bills you need to pay. Is someone you know in pain? Are you experiencing some form of diseases or unease? Name them. What are your feelings towards these issues? Don't let them dwell, but just recognize and enumerate them.

How do you feel about your body?

Without touching the body parts, focus your attention on just individual body parts. Focus your attention on your feet while it touches the ground. Notice the socks, and how they fit snugly on your foot. Notice your pants and how your legs contained in them. Notice your hips. Do you like your hips? Look at your stomach, do you like it? Notice your back. Feel the clothes on your back. How do you feel about your back? Notice every part of your face: the chin, the cheeks, your eyes, your ears, your nose, your eyebrows, your hair. How do you feel about your face?

What is your desire?

As you enter this program, what do you want to achieve the most? Do you want to lessen the bumps on your stomach? Do you want to have thinner cheeks? Do you want a broader back or whiter skin? Is this what you absolutely want? Is this really your heart's desire?

Do you want to move your body with more flexibility? Do you want to work more, spend more time with friends, and earn more? Do you want to breathe better? Do you want to live longer? Is this what you want? Is this your heart's desire?

Do you want to be healthy? Do you want to be healthy for yourself, for your family, for your loved ones? Is this what you really want? Is this really your heart's desire?

Do you want to change?

Finally, ask yourself, are you ready to change? Do you want to change? If no, then do not proceed. If at this point you feel not ready to make any changes in your life yet for some reason, then be at peace and continue as you are. But if you feel that you want to change your life, your way of eating and relating and you want to achieve your best self, then say, "Yes." Shout it in your mind and say, "Yes, I want to change." Say it repeatedly, over and over again. Form a mantra, "I want to change, I want to change, I want to change." Own it, command it, and make it your personal anthem.

Slowly, thank your body and tell it to help you. You will need to establish right relations with your body in order to change it. Breathe in and breathe out, breath in, breath out. Slowly, come out of the meditation.

Hopefully, this exercise could able you to commit to these mini-habits. The more you become aware and conscious of your behaviors, the more you can make a change in your life for the better. If you feel lost and disheartened, simply go back to this exercise and ground yourself once more to your goals. Remember that we are emphasizing on habits not just bursts of inspiration. By taking stock of yourself every now and then, you become more resolved in continuing these habits in your daily schedule.

I will outline you the seven habits for achieving a healthy lifestyle; bearing in mind our goal which is not only to lose weight but to achieve a healthy body and mind. This is not an exhaustive list; you can still think of your own. These are simple habits you can follow; which have been adopted by others and have proven effective. Remember that you can change your lifestyle one day at a time. It need not be as dramatic as a total overhaul because your body will be traumatized and won't cooperate. You simply should have the determination, resolve to continue and remain as healthy as you can. You can pick out one or two trips per day and apply them, see if it works for you and then continue doing it. Hopefully, the more you do it, the more it becomes automatic, and the body will respond easily.

Chapter 3: Eat Less, Eat Frequently, Eat Regularly

In general, we should watch what we are eating. If we want to target a sustained weight loss, we continue our binging lifestyle or eating whatever what is available. I am not recommending you to become a vegan overnight when it doesn't suit you. The last thing I would recommend is to stop eating. You should still eat, but you have to regulate what you eat and how much you eat. Dieticians are going to emphasize the quality of the food, the right combination of fats, proteins, lipids and other nutrient sources. But I would like to emphasize not just the quality and variety of foods you are going to eat, but also the quantity. If you are used to eating two cups of rice, maybe you can settle for one. If you are used to upsizing the order on fast foods, try going for the regular (or best, avoid fast food altogether). You have to train your body and your mind that you can survive on less. Load that less with the right nutrient sources, but you can manage with that less.

One way to trick your mind into eating less is to serve your food on small plates. If you've been to Japanese or a Korean restaurant, don't you feel frustrated that they always serve food on tiny plates? Well, all that has a purpose. If you have a large plate, the tendency for you is to fill that empty space with a lot of food. The space factor deceives you into getting more servings of potatoes or roast beef just so the plate could look full. If you use small plates, even just small portions already look full. You put a slab of steak on a tiny plate, and you wouldn't feel like finishing it up. Also, if you have smaller plates, you tend to slice food thinner into bite-sized pieces. This way, you can fit the food on the small plate. You don't want to see a mound of food packed to the brim. So smaller plates give you a delusion that you are eating a lot when in reality, you're not. When you look at Korean side dishes, they're all placed in small containers. It gives you the impression that you have a feast before you. But actually, you can all stack it in one plate. The delusion makes you achieve your health goals faster.

Usually, our breakfast, lunch, and dinner are full, heavy meals. Three times a day, our digestive system has to cope up with that workload of food. Three times a day, it will have to process big, bulky food by a combination of stomach juices, bile, lipases and other enzymes. What you can do to alleviate that stress is if you could space out the volume. Here, snacking works. Instead of three full meals, you can have five mini-meals in a day. Your breakfast can spread over two meals, your lunch and dinner could be halved so you could eat a snack in the afternoon. In this way, you are tricking your body that it is not constantly hungry, at the same time it doesn't need to work too much. Plus, it makes snacking legitimate!

When you eat, you should be regular in your meal times. Don't eat when you feel like it. Sometimes, you can get so engrossed in what you are doing that you tend to skip meals. That accounting report can be taken care off, but your stomach will cost you more if you don't take care of it. Your body should establish a certain pattern of releasing acids and receiving food. For example, you eat breakfast at around 7 AM. You do this regularly for one week. Your body will pick up the rhythm and prepare your stomach to release its digestive juices at that particular time. Imagine, if you don't have a regular meal time, your body will not know when to release digestive juices. If it has been used to receiving food for 7 AM and you fail to do so, it will still release the digestive juices, minus the food. These acids then hurt the lining of your stomach as a consequence. So the more you train your stomach to eat at a particular time, the more regular it will proceed with digestion, the less you hurt your linings.

Skipping meals is a no-no. When you skip a meal, you tend to compensate for it by eating more in the next meal. You feel starving, you will order more servings, and you overeat. If you compare regular meals with skipped meals, the volume of food is more for the latter. So we have to train our bodies to eat at particular times, even if we are not hungry. Sometimes, you feel that you are full already, but it's just lunch time. Eat anyway, however small. Your stomach will still release acids, so you better fill that thing up.

Chapter 4: Check the Label

Labels are there for a reason. They tell you how many calories there are for each serving of the food. In this way, you can compute the total number of calories you are eating. This process makes you more conscious of what you consume. Every food you take in has a corresponding caloric content, and you need to check the total calories you consume if you are going to push through with your diet plan. You can compare how much calories you if you consume a pack of cheese or nibble on crackers. By checking labels, you will know how much calories you can get from a serving of chips or a tub of ice cream. If you have a target caloric content for the day, reading the labels can help you decide what kinds of food to eat and what to ditch.

You also have to look out for other details aside from caloric content. You look at total fat and especially trans-fat content. This is very bad for your health because trans-fat is harder to digest. Food that has a lot of trans-fat includes cakes, biscuits, doughnuts, popcorn, butter, and cookies. All of these are so scrumptious and addicting. But they all have a lot of trans-fat that is not easily digestible. Go easy with the baked cakes, pies, cookies, biscuits, margarine, and doughnuts. They tend to be digested more slowly and stored longer, piling up in your belly. Too much of these can also cause certain diseases because they can block blood vessels leading to hypertension or heart attacks. So labels are there for a reason, so you use them.

By counting calories, you can make wise food decisions. You can even start bargaining with yourself. Suppose you like that delicious sugar-glazed doughnut on the nearest bakery. But you say you are only allowed 2,500 kilocalories per day. A regular doughnut will have 452 calories. You can allow yourself one doughnut, but you have to cut down on the other meals. You might have to give up that cup of rice or those two slices of bread. You can still eat what you want, but you have to maintain a range where the calories are still allowable for you. In this way, you are not completely depriving yourself. You just have to make various decisions on the sources of calories you can have for the day. Eating need not be a chore because you only have to eat oats for breakfast. If you eat oats every day, your palette can be desensitized, and you may not enjoy your food, even if it is the healthiest product in the world. Our body still needs a certain variety, an assortment of stimulation, rather than routine health bars. You can do that if you know where your calories are coming from and how you can vary where you source them.

Calorie counting can be a hassle. Especially if you hate Math or accounting, this exercise can throw you off back to your bad habits. Imagine, you go through your regular grocery shopping, and you have to stop now and then to check the label instead of dumping them all into the cart. This is effortful. But it is also rewarding once it becomes a habit. You become more conscious of the food you eat. You become more discerning between two similar products, say a sandwich spread or a tub of oil. They may accomplish the same purpose, but the calories will be way different. By counting calories, you are investing in yourself and your health.

Chapter 5: Goodbye Gadgets

I know you need to multitask. You have emails to answer, meetings you need to schedule and messages to reply. Millennials can do all these things all at once. Life becomes very easy when you have a mobile phone, plus a tablet, and a laptop with you. You are equipped with so many devices, and they can be pretty addicting. So you figure out that you can cut the time by eating while you work. In this way, you get your stomach full while at the same time, continuing to work. Is this ok? Wrong, very wrong. Not only it's poor etiquette especially if you are eating with other people, but it is downright unhealthy. You can get spaghetti sauces on your tablet, breadcrumbs on the keyboard or lemon juice on your phone. Your mind is bombarded by so many elements happening at the same time that it is unable to process each act individually. You need to take a break from your work. Just for 15 minutes, take your mind off the work so you could attend to your private business. Use it. You are not getting any richer if you give it up. So take a break.

Also, when you use a mobile phone or any electronic device when you eat, you are actually eating more than the usual. You get so engrossed in that show you are watching that you don't notice that you are eating extra servings of chips. You might have the first bite at the first minute of the hour, and the next could be at the last minute, and in a panic, you compensate by eating more. You feel hungry more, so you eat a lot. Or you could be very emotional when you are connected to your devices. You might be talking to an in-law, and in frustration, you could vent it out on the pizza. You might be watching a horror film, and between adrenaline scenes, you could be scooping more popcorn into security.

Plus, you don't chew very well when you are using a device. You are lazy to chew your food because you are focusing on the action on the screen. You might be talking too fast on the phone, or the series you are watching is nearing the finale. You don't notice that you just gulped that piece of steak whole or popped into a mouthful of cupcake. What does chewing do? Chewing is the first part of the digestive process. It manually breaks down the food into smaller pieces so that your enzymes have an easier time to act on the food. Chewing also allows more saliva to coat the food and start breaking down the starch content even before it reaches the stomach. If you swallow whole chunks of food, there is added stress to the esophagus, as the sheer amount moves down. The stomach will have a hard time breaking down the food into the acids. If the food stays longer in your body, your digestive system gets upset with the whole experience.

When you chew, you spent a long time savoring each bite. You begin to appreciate the food; not just experience it jamming your throat and disappearing from sight. It helps you bond with officemates or family or friends instead of your phone. Prolonged chewing can also prolong eating time, so you get fuller quickly. Your senses are more stimulated, so you are easily satiated. And this will help you eat less than your usual meal.

You can always return to your gadgets after the lunch break when you return to your work. They will always be there, ready at hand. But your health won't always be. So pay attention to your meal times and don't get too distracted by useless worrying and multi-tasking. Learn how to disconnect and enjoy your meal. Chew your food well.

Chapter 6: Emptying the Stash

We all have our secret stashes somewhere in the desk. There's a certain comfort in having food that is accessible. It is a safety net, a portable emergency cabinet, a quick fix. It's just addicting to put in a can of soda or a pack of Oreos or cheese crackers in your drawer for easy access. During a stressful bout, it's comforting to grab a quick energy booster or a sugary treat. It also makes sharing food also pretty easy. When somebody feels hungry, you just reach out from your secret stash and share away. In an office, sometimes there are designated people with the best stashes that everyone steals from legitimately.

But you know that if you are serious about your health goals, you have to empty that stash. And I mean completely empty. You need to stop sneaking into some secret hideout to get your sugar fix. That behavior is more appropriate if you are doing something illegal. Stop cheating yourself that it is only small, that you are not putting a whole meal in there. The smaller the snacks are, the easier it is to snatch one and empty it in your stomach. The presence of a secret stash lulls you into a false sense of security that is just going to widen that stomach.

And it's not going to easy, losing a safety net. The first few weeks of emptying your stash, you are going to compulsively reach out in your drawer and find an empty space. This is natural, and a good symbol of your commitment to health. The act of cleaning out your stash primes your brain that it is entering a new mode, a different lifestyle. Neurologically, when we get quick fixes, there are certain pathways in the brain that are stimulated. The more you do that particular pleasurable act, the more that pathway is strengthened. So when you reach out to your stash, that pathway is used more often than others. When you remove that act, the pleasure is immediately reduced. And your brain is not happy when it does not get that pleasure. It will want to return to that pleasure spot. But the trick is really to form new ways of achieving that pleasure without the weight gain.

Also, if you are hungry, you should still not have a secret stash. If you don't have that stash, you are going to be forced to stand up from your desk and go all the way to the cafeteria. You are going to wait in that queue of the elevator or worst you could end up exercising your way to the stairs. It will be such a hassle for you to go to the nearest snack bar, so you end up just forgetting about your hunger. Either way, you've tricked your mind again, and you're one step closer to your goals.

Or you could simply work or divert your attention to more productive things when you feel hungry in the middle of the day. It will be difficult at first because you have been used to getting instant fixes. But slowly, you will see that you can go through the day without a potato chip snack. You will notice that you can work longer or concentrate on meetings without having crutch crackers to back you up. It will take time, but you can train your body to not snack away. The brain is a malleable thing which will adapt to new situations if you give it time and effort. Appetites come and go, and they need not dictate to you when you should eat. You eat at the appropriate time, and not just when your brain tells you it wants its fix now.

Chapter 7: Don't Give in to Stress

You will always have stress. It comes up when you're working when you're with other people when you're alone. There are a lot of stressors out there that you don't need to make an effort to invent one. But you can cut on stresses that are not necessary. For example, if you are already late for work, then stop fretting already and think of the work after. If you have bills to pay, perhaps you can confront them after work, not during. If you lost a deal which you work hard for, focus on getting a new one instead of worrying about the past. You can allow yourself some time to mourn or take in the situation. But after some time, you have to bounce back and recover. There are stresses that we need to confront, but there are those we can let go.

We have to choose our stresses because it has an effect on our body. These useless anxieties cannot just be ignored because it has a manifestation of our behavior. Our body has a mechanism to confront the different stresses we experience. It is called the 'flight or fight' mode, a primitive way of interacting with a threatening stimulus. This mechanism releases a lot of adrenaline in the system when you are in a difficult situation. Your brain releases chemicals that pump you up so that you are ready to confront any immediate danger. This is good if you are suddenly in immediate danger. But if you don't need to confront anything immediately, this negatively impacts another system in the body. When you have the 'fight or flight' mode on, you are actually turning off the 'rest and digest' system. So when you are worrying while you are eating, your body is confused. It asks itself whether it wants to fight or digest the food. If you have a more serene disposition, worrying yourself unnecessarily, then your stomach will have a better time performing its functions.

When you also feel threatened or emotionally charged, you turn to food as a consolation, a safe spot. We see this, particularly in stress eating. After a long day at work, with so many tasks to do, so many people angry or agitating you, you normally feel a lot of stress. You want to alleviate that stress immediately, and there is a host of expressions for stress. If you are stressed, you can simply sleep it away, or find something relaxing such as music. When you have high levels of stress, you can turn into smoking or drinking which calms you down but hurts you in the longer run. You just want to address that negative impulse, NOW, in the immediate moment. And most of the time, food seems to be the natural recourse of stress.

Recall that when you are angry with a friend or a co-worker, you tend to have extra helpings of rice or anything filling. You see this most especially while you are trying to recall the event, such as talking about it with another friend. Or you are so sad after a heartbreak that you just want to be happy. You turn then to anything sweet. Chocolates, cookies, cake, anything that stimulates the endorphins makes you crave for more.

A study has even shown that binge-eating or hoard-eating is a response to running away from self-awareness. Heatherton and Baumeister (1991) found out that binge eaters often suffer from too much social pressure or expectations that they turn to eating. This removes them from thinking about their problems and what society thinks of them. What we see here is a problem that most of us have. Failure in the workplace or in school or in any relationship is deemed as an estimation of self-worth. When we fail, we think we did not live to a certain standard. So instead of confronting that feeling, we do not want to think and substitute the eating with it.

To assess whether the situation is worth your stress. You may not be able to control every circumstance or problem that comes up. But you can definitely change how you react to each situation. You can address it head on and confront it maturely. Don't abuse food and your body by giving in to the stress. Not only have you been beaten by the stress but you also begin to put on pounds on you. So the best way to fight back is to stand your ground, relax and let things unfold without you relying too much on food. Of course, there are days when the work is just difficult, and you just want to relax. Holidays and breaks are perfect for that. But you must always watch out for over-indulging yourself, feeling that you deserve that cake or you need that ice cream. You are worth more than that so don't go for cheap happiness. Elevate your taste and senses so you only crave for what will be good for your body.

Chapter 8: Hit the Kitchen

When you prepare your food, you tend to be more conscious of what you eat. You can see what you put in your dishes, whether it is the kind of oil you use or the amount of butter you sauté in. Most of us reason out that we don't have time. It is true, not all the time, but most of the time. We may be too preoccupied with work that we just want to order out pizza rather than cook our meals. The fast-food industry was built on that need. We have instant burgers, instant fries, instant chicken, instant noodles and instant everything. But we cannot just have "instant health" as much as we would like it to be. Most of these fast foods are darn tasty because the ingredients used are delicious but unhealthy. They contain a lot of calories and fats which you forget in between bites of a juicy cheeseburger sandwich or tasty hash browns. Fast food brings us convenience and flavor at the price of our health.

When you cook your food, you become responsible for what you eat. You begin to see just how much oil you are using, the amount of salt you sprinkle, the sugar you mix in. When you just order food, you just remain at the level of the taste. But you eat it without actually knowing what went into that food. You don't have control over what they actually put in there. You just know that it has chicken and some vegetables. You don't know if they cooked it canola or in olive oil, you don't know if they used a special seasoning. And you're just sitting down. Or that doughnut must be very delicious, but when you calculate just how much calories you get from a piece, you'd be shocked. Cooking somehow makes calorie counting more controlled and managed and doable.

The process of preparing the food is in itself rewarding. You are able to make dishes come alive with your own hands. It takes an effort to prepare food: peeling the vegetables, rinsing them, washing dishes, chopping, slicing, sautéing, boiling, frying and plating. There is such a long process you still need to go before you can eat. In the process, you are already being satiated. And while you are cooking, you are already tasting. When you are the cook, you usually eat less because you have already eaten the food beforehand, many times over. Cooking is such a rewarding experience, especially if you are cooking for other people. Cooking bonds people together, as they criticize and appreciate your work.

It is not true that not everyone can cook. Not everyone would want to try cooking. They would rather eat food that has been made without their effort. You might reason out that you are no good as a cook or that you don't know how. Maybe, you just haven't given it a try or the best effort you can. Or you are always comparing yourself to Michelin restaurants. The comparison is quite off because you are setting too high a standard for yourself. There are very simple meals you can cook in a short time, that don't even require expensive equipment. There are quick meals you can whip up without taking your time from sleep or overtime work. The operative word here is to "Try." Try first before you complain. Try cooking. Try baking. Try reading a recipe or watching a video. Try for your health. Try to cook for others and see how they'll react. Not only would you become conscious of the contents of your food, but you would gain a necessary life skill.

It is also true that if you cook your own meals, you can save a lot more. When you eat out, the food you order is not really worth what you eat. The price you pay the restaurant covers the fee of the servers, of the company, of the expenses in the equipment, procurement of the food, preparation, serving, advertising, the whole works. Sometimes, you are paying more for the venue and the ambiance rather than the food itself. When you cook your own food, you take out the middlemen like the cooks and the waiters and the managers. You get to keep your money, learn a life skill and get filled up for half the cost of a normal classy restaurant. You lose weight, and you save up on the money.

Chapter 9: Walk, Walk, Walk

If you don't have time to go to the gym or do any workout, walking is probably the most inexpensive workout you can do. These fitness clubs entice you to join their program for a month in exchange for instant weight loss while burning a hole in your wallet. You have to buy clothes and equipment for some programs. You buy into this, but after a while, you cannot sustain it and drop out. Or for those who want to spend less or want to exercise from home, they try to buy fitness equipment or machines. This is optimal for those who cannot visit the gym regularly. But, it can be dangerous if you don't know how to use these machines and weights well. They can damage your body in the long run if you fail to use them appropriately. And some of this equipment is insanely expensive. You need to have an area in your house to stock them and keep them from rusting or wearing down.

You have to find creative ways of walking such as taking the flight of stairs instead of the elevator. You can drop your car somewhere far from your office, so you still need to walk some distance. When you are going to eat, choose a place that is farther than usual it will force you to walk. It is effortful, but you need that kind of effort for your health. Imagine, for the next eight to ten hours you will be stuck in that seat because you are concentrated on your work. This is not good because a sedentary lifestyle can predispose you to certain diseases involving the blood circulation. You get less oxygen and nutrients in your body by remaining in one position for a long time. Try pacing up and down your office aisle once in a while just to stimulate your circulation.

The kind of walking you should take is the kind that will make you sweat. This is different from a leisurely walk which will stretch your muscles. When you sweat while you walk; you are making your heart pump faster, your circulation to flow better and your breath deeper. If you just stroll in the park to work, then you achieve none of that. Plus, walking can save a lot of money for you. It consumes no electricity or gas while achieving the same distance by walking.

It would be good for you if you had a companion walking with you. It could be a health-conscious officemate. It could be a friend who happens to take the same routine as you. Whatever the circumstance may be, another person walking can motivate you to keep on walking. Just the simple presence of another being can make you walk faster. The walk will be long, but if you are with somebody you like, then the journey would not be as painful or as noticeable as you think it will be. If you feel like giving up, the other person can help you bounce back from your negativity. They can silence your inner critique. Their presence tells you that you are not alone in this endeavor to live a healthy life. You are going to be healthy, thanks to the encouragement of others.

Conclusion

There is a saying that you need two weeks or so to form a habit. You have to regularly perform a task for the two weeks until your brain changes its neuronal networks and strengthens the pathways of the new behavior. After the two weeks, the habit becomes automatic that you do without consciously thinking about doing it. The habit becomes part of you that you no longer struggle with the decision of doing or not, you just do it. And this is the goal of this book. You have to follow the seven tips on weight loss faithfully for the next two or four weeks. It will be very difficult during the first week as the body is still adapting to the changes. But after the first week, you will begin to be more relaxed and receptive to these habits. You can notice small changes in your body size or disposition. If you keep this up, you can even reach your desired body size without much effort. Nothing is impossible with the brain. You just have to master it, to train it, to motivate it to achieve what you want which is to become healthier.

Hopefully, these mini-habits are doable for you. I call them mini because they are not too obtrusive actions that you can drastically change your life. Those programs that offer a 90-degree turn from your current lifestyle are bound to fail because they are interesting only during the first week. After a while, people can get tired and bored with these routines they would slump back to their old habits. These mini-habits are meant to replace your old bad habits. For example, if you tend to snack a lot, I tell you to empty your secret stash. The snacking can be ingrained in your system, something you always look for. But you can remove these habits by replacing with the new ones. You want to form new networks in your brain, ones that are more supportive of your desire to lose weight.

All these tips are designed for you to trick your mind and body into a healthier lifestyle. Choose what works for you the best, but by my experience; all of these works. Losing weight and choosing a healthy lifestyle is strenuous. You cannot fit in your pants by continuing your mindless lifestyle. If we become more conscious of our actions, we can strike out unhealthy eating patterns and develop good habits. Remember that your goal is not just to lose weight, but to have a healthy life, for yourself and your loved ones. You can only accomplish this through mindful thinking. Master your mind, and you can master your body. One mini-habit at a time.

-- Kyle J. Benson

Check Out Other Books

Go here to check out other books that might interest you:

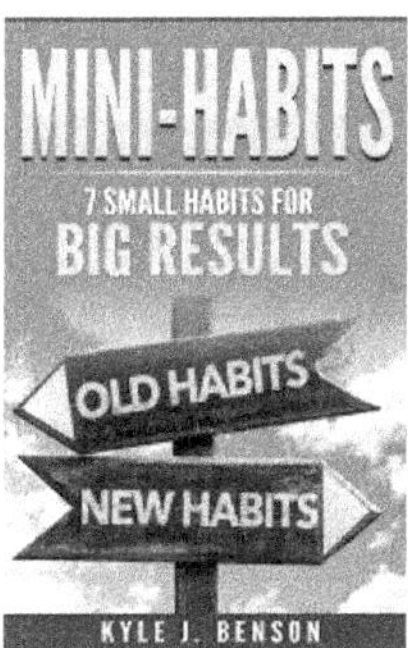

Mini-Habits: 7 Small Habits for Big Results
https://www.amazon.com/dp/B077FC1YGS

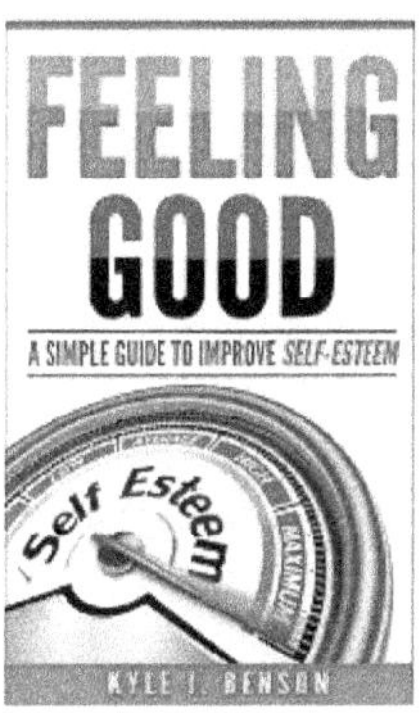

Feeling Good: A Simple Guide to Improve Anxiety

https://www.amazon.com/dp/B077P6CGZL

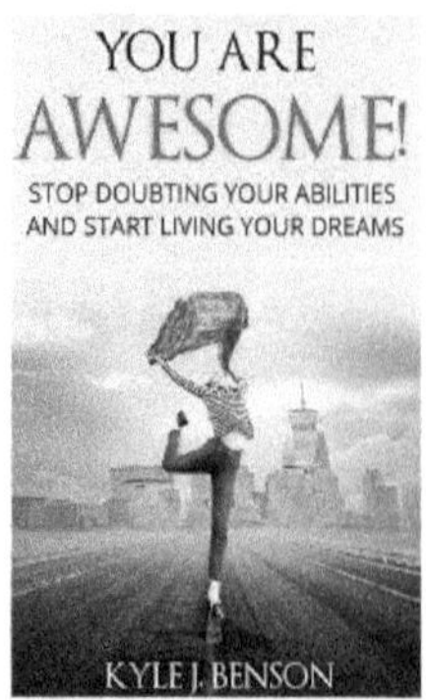

You Are Awesome!: Stop Doubting Your Abilities and Start Living Your Dreams

https://www.amazon.com/dp/B077TGG7F7

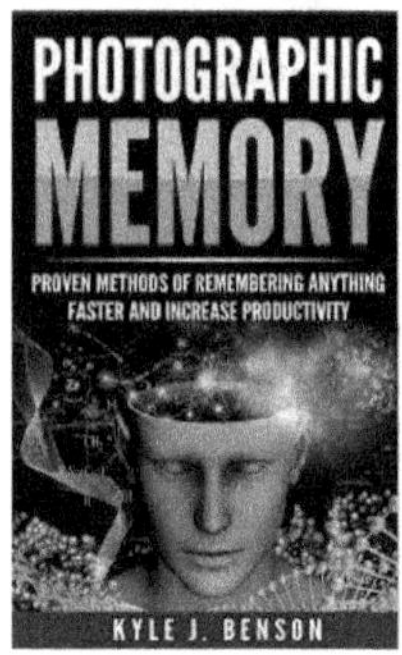

Photographic Memory: Proven Methods of Remembering Anything Faster and Increase Productivity

https://www.amazon.com/dp/B077VTXQ76